Poop Faster
with a Deep Breath

M.T. Colon

Copyright

Poop Faster with a Deep Breath
Copyright © 2024 by M.T. Colon
ISBN: 979-8-3448-0496-5

First Edition

Proudly Printed in the USA

Legal Disclaimer
This book is intended solely for educational and informational purposes. It is not a substitute for medical advice, diagnosis, or treatment. The techniques and suggestions provided in this book should not be performed without consulting a qualified

healthcare professional, especially if you have any preexisting medical conditions or concerns.

The author and publisher make no representations or warranties concerning the accuracy or completeness of the information in this book and expressly disclaim any liability for any injuries, losses, or damages incurred by individuals who choose to apply the information herein. By using this book, you agree to assume full responsibility for any consequences resulting from following its content.

Warning

Some techniques described in this book involve physical exertion and may pose health risks if performed incorrectly or too forcefully. Proceed with caution, especially during techniques that involve breath control or muscle engagement. Stop immediately if you experience any pain, discomfort, or adverse effects, and seek medical attention if necessary.

Attempting these methods is entirely at your own risk. Always use caution and practice slowly, particularly with any steps that recommend a specific breathing technique. Failure to follow these guidelines may result in injury. Results may vary, and the techniques may not be suitable for all individuals.

This book is a work of nonfiction, and while the author has made every effort to ensure accuracy, no guarantee is provided that the techniques will work as described for every individual.

Contents

1 Introduction   1

2 The Method: Breathing DOWN and BACK   3

3 Step-by-Step Guide # 1   5

4 Step-by-Step Guide # 2   11

5 What if you're still struggling?   15

6 Conclusion   17

1

Introduction

Your cute toddler is drawing on the walls. Your phone in the other room is ringing. Your dog is barking. And you...you...are stuck on the toilet. Again. Helplessly waiting. For that stool to take its time. To come out. This book dives straight into practical steps to help you eliminate stools faster. Much, much faster. So you can get back out there. Pick up your toddler. Answer your phone. Grab the dog. Take charge of your life and everything else that needs you.

2

The Method: Breathing DOWN and BACK

Your mother told you pushing your poop out is bad for you. That's why you sit patiently and wait. But that's only when you push by straining. There's another way. Push using your DIAPHRAGM which is also known as BREATHING. It works by expanding your lungs against your diaphragm against your intestines to push your stools out. But achieving this simple idea is not so easy. That's what this book is for. Your lungs can expand in many directions, up, sideways, and most importantly DOWN and BACK. By breathing down and back, your lungs will push your diaphragm against your intestines, speeding up elimination. Here's why it works and how to start:

3

Step-by-Step Guide # 1

There's two different ways for you to train your body on how to breath to poop. Here's the first way, it's safer and easier, but requires more will power and organization skills:

Step 1: Breathing

Take a breath in and out. Which part of your body moves—chest, shoulders, stomach, back? Most people expand their lungs horizontally through their shoulders and chest. Instead, our goal is a slight expansion in our lower back. Here's how to get there:

1. Lie on a hard surface, like your floor, on your back.

2. Close your eyes to focus on the feeling. And minimize your breathing to focus on the muscle contraction.

3. Breathe DOWN towards your butt, directing the airflow DOWN and toward your BACK.

Indicators You're Doing It Right:

- Your lower back expands with air

- Your intestines feel uncomfortable pressure

- You may pass gas

- Your chest and belly stay still

- Internally, your lungs move down and back

- You take 10s to fill your lungs

Indicators You're Doing It Wrong:

- Your ribcage expands out

- Your belly goes out

- You take less than 10 seconds to fill your lungs

Once you can consistently breath DOWN and BACK in 10 seconds, it's time to try forcing out a fart with your breathing. YOU MUST DO IT IN NO FEWER THAN TEN SECONDS OTHERWISE YOU COULD DAMAGE YOUR ANUS. This technique is powerful, I have damaged myself with it, so please, start slow.

Step 2: Farting

Farts are like a practice stool, but much safer as they're just gas, you won't damage your anus.

1. When you feel gas, breathe in deeply and slowly, remember, ten seconds, using the DOWN and BACK method.

2. Notice how the gas is pushed out and expelled quickly. You'll appreciate how powerful it is.

Once you get used to expelling farts with your breathing, and you're good at controlling the speed, you're ready for live fire.

Step 3: Pooping

With the breathing technique mastered, and practice gained, you're ready to try this on live rounds:

- When you're on the toilet ready to go, take a deep, slow ten second breath.

- Inhale, DOWN, and BACK.

- You should feel yourself pushing the stool gently by your body as the pressure builds up inside of you from the power of your breath.

- STOP at any point if anything feels uncomfortable. If you stop breathing, the pressure will also stop and your stool will slow down.

- As you exhale the stool will no longer be pushed, relax and let the stool process continue naturally.

- Avoid contracting your anus as much as you can as that can pinch the stool which can make it more difficult to pass the stool. But if you have to, you have to.

- Take it slow, especially if the stool is hard as that can be rough on your body.

Step 4: Managing Your Anal Contraction Reflex

When you push with your diaphragm long enough, which can happen with longer stools, eventually your body will want to contract. Try to avoid this as long as you can, contracting your anus can pinch a stool half way. Pinching a stool is slow. It's a second half, which can be a pain to get out. To train the reflex, just keep fighting it. Eventually your body will naturally fight it and you'll go longer and longer without the contraction, eventually going the whole bowel movement without having it.

4

Step-by-Step Guide # 2

However, you might find it difficult to stay motivated. If so,
then we'll do it live.

Step 1: Put book in bathroom

Put this book in your bathroom. Right now. You can finish reading it next time you're on the toilet. Did you put it there? Good. It'll remind you to do this EVERY TIME YOU POOP. It is important to have a reminder to practice the technique.

Step 2: Do It Live

When you're passing a stool the book will remind you to do it live. So, Do It Live. No practice rounds. No dry runs. No lying down. No farting. Just. Do. It. But remember, GO SLOW (10s per inhale) or you could damage your anus. Trying this way also gives you a bit more feedback because when you do it right you'll immediately feel your stool being pushed out faster and when you do it wrong you won't. Easy feedback and easy motivation. You're reminded when to do it, and if you do it right, you'll get instant feedback and instant reward. And the important thing at the end of the day is that you do it, and poop faster, right?

5

What if you're still struggling?

Diaphragm breathing is hard. Don't give up. But, I did it, and so can you. You can poop faster. Finding a poop coach is a bit embarrassing. But! Generic "Diaphragm Breathing" is not. you can find help from any local voice coach. But be firm, you don't want regular 'belly breathing' where your stomach goes in and out. You want specifically your lungs to push DOWN and BACK to push your intestines (against your stools). Explain this clearly and that you want hands on feedback where they can feel where your lungs are going. So they can tell where your lungs are going and where they should be instead.

6

Conclusion

By mastering DOWN and BACK breathing, you'll be able to speed up bowel movements. When your toddler starts drawing, you won't be helplessly waiting. You'll be right there to pick him back up into your arms. When your boss calls, you'll be right there to pick up the phone. And when the dog starts barking, you can give him a nice head scratch to remind him how much you love him. And you'll get your life back.